Yoga for Beginners

Daily Guide of Basic Yoga for Beginning Students

(Private Yoga Lessons Series)

Michelle Nicole

Yoga for Beginners

Daily Guide of Basic Yoga for Beginning Students

(Private Yoga Lessons Series)

Disclaimer

All the information included in this book has been carefully researched and checked for accuracy.

The reader assumes the risk and full responsibility for all actions, and the author will not be held responsible for any loss or damage, whether consequential, incidental, special or otherwise that may result from the information presented in this publication.

I have relied on my own experience as well as different sources to write this book, and I have done my best to check facts and to give credit where it is due.

Thank you for understanding.

Table of Contents

Introduction to the World of Yoga

Each body is a universe; as good a universe as you could conceive ~ Swami Amar Jyoti

Hi there, my name is Michelle and I am a living, breathing witness of the beautiful art that is yoga and the wonderful benefits it provides an individual. My life has positively changed on many levels since I started practicing yoga many years ago.

Through this book, I want to share with you my knowledge about yoga and help you transform your life for the good as well.

This book is intended for individuals who want to know more about yoga and its practice, those who are looking for a healthy change in their life, and those who simply want to be at peace with their mind and body.

Why Practice Yoga?

I cannot fathom how to begin answering this question. Personally, I got into yoga simply because I was stressed from my job and wanted an activity to help me take my mind off my worries. But, as time passed, I realized that yoga was doing much more to my mind and body than I had ever expected.

Sure, I could give you countless reasons why you should practice yoga – to lose weight, to improve your flexibility and strength, to sharpen your focus and concentration, to start a healthy lifestyle, to attain spiritual development - the list goes on.

Yoga can indeed provide these benefits, but getting to know this art form on a deeper level and understanding its real purpose will open doors for you that you didn't know existed.

The word YOGA comes from the Sanskrit word yuji which means to connect or unite, The term 'wholeness' is etymologically related to the words healthy and holy.

Through yoga, you will be able to develop a clear mind, a healthy body, and a free spirit – and unite them all into a whole, which is needed to survive the chaos of a world we live in today.

So why practice yoga? Because you know in the back of your mind that you are meant to be whole in every sense of the word.

How to Use this Book

In this book I have detailed the basic concepts of yoga, how to get ready for practicing yoga, the benefits of yoga, the best yoga warm-up exercises, basic postures, breathing and meditation techniques, and so much more!

As a beginning yogi, allow this book to help you experience the wonders of yoga and create a positive change in your life today.Let this book be your guide as you open your mind, body, and spirit to the world of yoga where you can truly flourish.

I'm excited to begin, are you?

Yoga Basics

I believe that you can't truly embrace a practice without understanding it first. So, in this chapter we will discuss the basics of yoga, its history, what it is and what it is not, plus the many wonderful benefits you can gain from practicing it regularly.

A Brief History of Yoga

Although the subject has been researched for over a century now, no one has been able to pinpoint the earliest beginnings of yoga. Scholars have linked the practice to Stone Age Shamanism where religious mediators aim to heal community members through improving their human condition. In its earliest form, yoga was a community-oriented practice, as opposed to the yoga we know today.

Early on, yoga was thought to have originated about the same time Buddhism was founded (500 B.C.); but, in the 1920's, archeologists discovered the Indus Civilization, the largest in early antiquity. Excavators found yogi-like figures engraved on soapstone seals in the ruins of the cities Harappa and Mohenjo Daro. The stones date back to 3,000 B.C. and are considered to be the first archeological evidence of the existence of yoga.

This supports the opinion of experts who are sure that yoga originated from India more than 5,000 years ago.

Initially, it focused on applying and understanding the world, but later the focus shifted to self-enlightenment.

The history of yoga can be divided into four periods: the Vedic Period, the Pre-Classical Period, the Classical Period and the Post-Classical Period.

The Vedic Period is characterized by the existence of the Vedas, a sacred scripture that contains a collection of hymns that praise a divine being. The Vedas contains the earliest yogic teachings (Vedic Yoga) which show ceremonies and rituals that aim to surpass the mind's limitations.

The Pre-Classical Period is marked by the creation of the Upanishads, 200 scriptures that discuss the Brahman (ultimate reality), the atman (transcendental self) and the relationship between these two concepts.

During this period yoga was also found to have similarities with Buddhism which focuses on the importance of physical poses and meditation. In 500 B.C., the oldest known yoga scripture, Bhagavad-Gita (Lord's Song) was created.

The Classical Period is marked by the creation of Patanjali's Yoga Sutra in the 2nd century. An attempt to define Classical Yoga, the creation contains about 195 sutras and stressed on the Eight Limbs of Classical Yoga, which are:

- Asanas (physical pose or exercise)
- Dharana (focus and concentration)
- Dhyana (meditation)
- Niyama (personal observation of purity, study and tolerance)
- Pranayama (controlled breathing and breath regulation)
- Pratyahara (withdrawal of the senses to prepare for meditation)
- Samadhi (ecstasy)
- Yama (ethical values)

The Post-Classical Period is characterized by the spread of yoga literature and practice. It is different from the previous periods as it encourages an individual to accept the reality and live in the moment as opposed to liberating oneself from reality, which the first three periods focused on.

In the early 19th century, yoga was introduced to the West. Maharishi Mahesh popularized Transcendental Meditation in the 1960's. About the same time, a yoga guru named Swami Sivananda introduced his modified Five Principles of Meditation, which are:

- Asanas (proper exercise)

- Dhyana (positive thinking and meditation)
- Pranayama (proper breathing)
- Savasana (proper relaxation)
- Proper Diet

What Yoga Is and Isn't

We live in a time where diets and weight loss methods are the craze; so, it is not surprising that many people who practice yoga are unaware of its true purpose. As a result, there are large numbers of people who practice yoga for the wrong reasons; and I don't want you to be one of them.

You cannot expect to achieve a right outcome from a wrong intention; and practicing yoga is no exception.

What Yoga Is

Yoga sees the human body as a temple and treats it with utmost care and respect. Yoga is an ancient discipline that must be understood, practiced, and mastered to become an effective tool that allows you to function efficiently in all aspects

The entire yoga system is based on three primary structures: Breathing, Meditation and Exercise.

The various breathing and meditation techniques aim to develop a strong sense of s.elf-awareness by re-connecting an individual to his/her inner self. Through this, one will be able to experience calmness, relaxation, and clarity of the mind.

The exercises and poses incorporated in yoga are intended to put pressure on different areas of the body for increased health and efficiency.

What Yoga Isn't

As I mentioned earlier, many people misunderstand the true goals of yoga. To help you understand the discipline, you must know that yoga is NOT any of the following:

1. **An aerobic exercise meant to sculpt the body or help with weight loss**. Yoga is not meant to feed the vanity or ego. It is, first and foremost, a meditation practice meant to calm the mind in order to discover your true self. Toning the body and losing weight should be considered a by-product yoga.

2. **About flexibility.** Yoga is primarily about practicing balance and accepting who you are as a person – it wrong to practic yoga to become flexible.

   The poses are designed to eventually calm the mind, which should be your primary purpose of practicing this art. Doing this, you promote harmony and peace in your entire being. Flexibility of the body comes as a result of constant practice of poses that are meant to calm your inner being.

3. **Practicing yoga exists only during a session**. Yoga should be considered a way of life. Every thing

you do in your daily life, every connection with a fellow being is also a yoga moment.Therefore, yoga is a practice that will help you achieve clarity of thought and a peaceful mind.

4. **A religion or cult.** This is not true. How to practice yoga can't be found in a single guide book or a Bible. The teachings of each yogi master are developed according to their respective experience, their body's range of motion and qualities, bodily limits, and spiritual growth. Blindly following any teaching is not wise and can very likely create setbacks that you will have to overcome. This is because teachers, no matter how experienced, are still mere humans.

5. **Merely about poses.** When practicing yoga, the poses are considered meditation in movement. By moving while meditating you are freeing your breath to experience a clear mind as you execute each pose. Still, yoga poses don't need to be in a specific form. It is more like finding which position is most comfortable for you so you can stay still for meditation. However, regardless of how many poses you master, if you have a mind that is filled with negativity, you are not practicing yoga, but merely executing the poses.

Benefits of Yoga

Yoga has remarkable effects on each individual. It is very effective in the synchronization of the mind, body, and spirit for the attainment of inner peace and harmony.

Stress has an impact on all systems in the body. Stress from personal conflicts tends to weigh down an individual and greatly affect all personal and work relationships, daily performance, and general interaction with society.

Yoga can help correct these problems.

Below is a list of specific benefits that can be derived from the practice of yoga:

1. **Increased lubrication of tendons, joints, and ligaments.** Yoga positions focus on the development of specific ligaments and tendons.Different poses affect different joints of the body. This includes parts that are not touched through standard exercises.

2. **Increased Flexibility** Studies show that even people who have never exercised will experience a remarkable increase in flexibility with constant practice of yoga – including parts of the body that are not usually the focus of any exercise program..

3. **Massages every organ in the body.** Yoga is the only practice known to thoroughly work all internal organs of the body, including the ones that barely get stimulated under normal circumstances.

4. **Total body detoxification.** In addition to organ massage, yoga also stimulates blood flow, which assists in total body detoxification.

   With regular yoga practice, you will notice a dramatic increase in zest and energy, plus the added benefit of delayed ageing and much more.

5. **Very effective for mental relaxation.** Yoga practice trains a person to relax.This includes learning to calm the mind, to enjoy self-acceptance, and to think positive thoughts.The more you practice yoga, the more effective you will be in handling stressful situations.

6. **Enhances physical appearance.** Many people who practice yoga develop a strong, toned, and flexible body. Since it efficiently enhances the metabolism, you experience increased vitality and energy. Yoga is also known to relieve pain.

7. **Increased spiritual awareness.** Regular yoga practice will help you develop an increased sense of awareness, because it merges the spirit, mind, and body. As a result, you become more sensitive to your feelings and your body, to people around you, and much more. As your awareness grows, you will begin to eliminate the negativities in your life, which results in an incredible feeling of calmness.

Getting Ready to Practice Yoga

With some background information in place, you are now ready to begin your practice of the discipline. I know you are psyched to begin (I am, too!); but, before we start there are a few more things you should know.

Who Can and Can't Practice Yoga

Bryan Kest, a well-known yoga instructor in Southern California, said, "If you can breathe, you can practice yoga!"

Anyone – young or old, fit or supple, can practice yoga. It is a non-competitive discipline in which each individual works within his/her own level of comfort.

As a point of information, there is some controversy regarding the safety of practicing yoga in certain situations, which I had addressed below.

I have expressed my opinion on each point, but if you have questions, please do your own research before continuing.

Yoga During Pregnancy

Many yoga advocates firmly believe that pregnant women can safely perform yoga. In fact, it is widely accepted that the right kind of yoga can be beneficial to their health.

As we all know, pregnancy is often accompanied by a plethora of discomforts such as nausea, sleeplessness, irritability, shortness of breath, lower back pain, leg cramps... the list goes on. As amazing as it is, prenatal yoga can help reverse many of these issues.

Prenatal yoga involves gentle stretching that moves various parts of the body such as the neck and the arms, which helps relieve lower back pain and leg cramps. The breathing techniques practiced in prenatal yoga can help alleviate shortness of breath and prepares the woman for contractions during labor.

Meditation techniques will help with focus and concentration, preventing anxiety and stress as well as preventing sleeplessness and irritability.

Finally, prenatal yoga incorporates safe poses that will enhance muscle strength, flexibility, and endurance, all of which are important during labor and delivery.

Of course, as with any activity you choose to do when pregnant, it is vital that you take precautions. When you attend a prenatal yoga class, be sure to inform your instructor that you are pregnant and the trimester you are in. This will help your instructor monitor your poses for safety considerations when doing certain asanas (body positions).

For example, asanas that are done on your back are not safe after the first trimester because they can decrease blood flow to the uterus. After the second trimester, your center of gravity will start to shift, so it is recommended that you do standing asanas with your heels to the wall to avoid losing your balance.

Safe yoga poses for pregnant women include the Butterfly Stretch, the Cat-Cow Pose, the Cobra Pose, Seated Forward Bend, Standing Forward Bend and the Triangle Pose. Backbends, Headstands, Handstands, the Camel Pose, and the Upward Bow. Any inversion is strictly prohibited for pregnant women.

Yoga During Menstruation

Some believe that women should stop practicing yoga completely during their periods, while others believe that it helps alleviate menstrual problems..

The menstrual cycle is delicate – it is reflected in a woman's mental and physical state of well-being. That is why safe postures accompanied by breathing and meditation techniques will benefit a woman during her period.

Menstruation is actually a period of heightened awareness and sensitivity, making it a perfect time to connect with your inner self through yoga.

The important thing is to listen to your body during your period. Every woman is different; so, it is important to pay attention to your intuition and do what you think your body needs at that time. Your body can help you decide whether yoga is a good idea, or not.

During heavy days of your period, experts do not recommend certain asanas such as forearm balances, hand balances, headstands, shoulder stands and other postures that promote blood flow. Focus on breathing exercises or simple postures that will not make you uncomfortable.

Yoga When Recovering from Muscle or Skeletal Injury

Contrary to popular belief, those who are suffering from muscle or skeletal injury can indeed perform yoga. Yoga is a good activity for both the muscles and the bones, even on occasions of injury, where directed by a certified instructor.

The movement from asanas to asanas requires slow, deep stretching which opens up the muscles to allow enhanced detoxification and blood flow.

Also, most people are shallow breathers, which yoga can correct through the breathing techniques. Shallow breathing deprives the muscles of oxygenated and nutrient-rich blood which is vital for their optimum function and recovery.

Yoga also relaxes specific natural reflexes called spinal reflexes which cause muscle contraction.

These spinal reflexes are:

1. **The Myotatic Reflex (Stretch Reflex)**Thiis is when a lengthened muscle automatically tenses up when put in a stretched position.Through yoga breathing techniques and meditation, this reflex can be stopped by decreasing inflammation and pain, allowing an injured muscle to stretch with ease.

2. **The Inverse Myotatic Reflex** will respond when an asanas is held for about 12-15 seconds. This is beneficial for any injured muscle because it allows a group of stretched muscles to relax. This is also helpful when dealing with muscle spasms.

3. **The Reciprocal Relaxation Reflex** causes a group of shortened muscles to tense up. Yoga can reverse this by relaxing the group of muscles and stretching various muscles in the body including injured ones that are difficult to reach such as tiny back muscles and rib muscles.

Practicing yoga can also be beneficial in cases of skeletal injury. Some yoga classes are tailored for bone recovery, building bone strength, and improving osteoporosis.

These special classes combine adaptive asanas and therapeutic exercises from Pilates and physical therapy. They work by incorporating breathing exercises during the inflammation phase - followed by a period of slow, gentle stretching, and a series of non-complex asanas to help in recovery.

NOTE OF CAUTION: When you're suffering from muscle or skeletal injury, be sure to seek the advice of a medical expert to ensure it is safe to practice yoga.

Starting Your First Yoga Session

Your first yoga session can make you feel both anxious and excited. I remember my first time stepping into a yoga studio. I was experiencing butterflies in my stomach; but, I felt like I was where I was supposed to be. Little did I know that day would change my life forever and here I am, a yoga advocate many years later.

One important thing to consider when attending a yoga class for the first time is your attire. The discipline is all about focusing on control, calmness, and flexibility. It is important to dress appropriately so that what you wear will not get in the way of achieving these goals.

What to Wear

For a typical yoga workout, wearing a fitted or semi-fitted tee, camisole, halter top or tank top is ideal. While a baggy shirt may seem the most comfortable, it is not ideal when doing inverted poses.

As for bottoms, a quick-dry capri or full-length pants is recommended. Steer clear of bottoms that have a drawstring waist because it will interfere with asanas that require you to lie on the floor face down. Avoid any type of bottom garment that restricts your movement. Also, be sure that the pant length is appropriate to avoid tripping.

The discipline is typically practiced barefoot; but, if you want to increase your traction; or if you are worried about hygiene, you can opt to wear shoes with bendable soles, strappy foot thongs, or yoga socks (socks with individual toes).

Yoga-specific clothing makes use of biodegradable or organic fibers which are soft, stretchy and effective moisture-absorbers. If you don't have access to clothing made specifically for yoga, any type of athletic clothing that meets the above-specified criteria will do.

During cold weather you can also opt for layering. You can wear lightweight zip-up hoodies or long-sleeved thermal hoodies to help loosen your muscles, raise your core temperature, and prevent chills that will interfere with concentration.

Also, you have to take into consideration the type of yoga you are practicing. If you want to practice power yoga or Bikram yoga, it is ideal that you wear a sports bra and shorts because you will be sweating a lot.

Duration of a Yoga Session

While a typical yoga class lasts for 1½ hours, the length of a session depends on various factors such as the type and level of yoga you are practicing and the goals you want to achieve through your workout.

For example, some meditation sessions could be completed in only 20 minutes. Advanced sessions usually last longer, (2 hours or so) performing breathing techniques, chanting, meditation, and asanas.

Every yoga session includes three main phases: Purva Anga (preparation), Pradhana Anga (core phase) and Uttara Anga (conclusion phase). Each yoga workout should also have a warm-up and a cool-down. Warm-up exercises will prepare the body for yoga; while cool-down exercises will bring the body down to rest.

In most cases, it is not unusual to become enthusiastic when starting out with yoga. In the beginning, you are keen to put extra effort to learn the program. However, bear in mind that yoga will involve investing lot of effort and patience on your part. It is an intense program which requires constant practice to perfect. Be patient with yourself and with the learning process.

Tips Before Starting Your First Session

- Take time to practice the basic asanas. These include Downward-Facing Dog, Upward-Facing Dog, Warrior 1 and 2 etc. Practicing will help you become more comfortable with the poses during the first day of your first yoga session.

- Make sure that you have your yoga gear ready.

- To avoid any inconveniences during your yoga workout, make sure to empty your bladder and bowels. Make it a point to observe this habit before attending every yoga session.

- Avoid any food intake approximately 2 hours prior to your yoga class. This is to keep you from feeling heavy and tired during the session. If you have to eat something, go for a light snack.

- Bring only a water bottle, a towel, a change of clothes. and yoga props to a session. Refrain from bringing your cellphone, tablet, or anything that could interfere with concentration.

- Don't expect to perfect the various breathing techniques or asanas on the first day. Some take years to master a pose. Just breathe, relax, and enjoy yourself.

Types of Yoga Recommended for Beginners

Since there are many types of yoga, you may be wondering which type would be most suitable for you. There are many different opions on this question; but,no definite answer because every person's needs are different and you must decide what you need.

As a beginner it is important to choose a yoga type that is appropriate for your health condition, fitness level, physical endurance capability, and spiritual objective.

If you have not been physically active in the past, start with a slower and gentler type of yoga. Obviously, you have to go through the basics first in order to build up endurance and flexibility, which are developed over time with constant yoga practice.

Listed below are different types of yoga that are recommended for beginners. Use this list to help you determine which one will be the best choice for you as a starting point.

Iyengar Yoga

This is one of the best types of yoga for beginners. The primary focus of this type of yoga is on the proper alignment and precise movement of the body. Beginners are advised to use accessories for support, like straps and blocks. This is to avoid injuries and enable you to comfortably execute different poses.

Because of the flexible pose modifications involved with Iyengar Yoga, people who constantly experience neck and back pain will benefit greatly from it.

With constant practice, this will also remedy bad posture since it primarily focuses on proper body alignment.This type will also expose you to classic yoga poses and postures, which means that you will also be learning the basic fundamentals of the other yoga styles.

Hatha Yoga

This is another type of yoga well-suited for beginners. Hatha is considered the all-around yoga style, because it primarily focuses on blending relaxation, breathing exercises, meditation, and poses. Simply put, the core elements of yoga are combined and thoroughly covered which makes Hatha a great foundation for yoga beginners.

Bikram Yoga

Also referred to as hot yoga, Bikram Yoga is performed in an extremely warm room. The heat helps in stretching tissues since heat itself is known to effectively loosen muscles, this type of yoga efficient for increasing flexibility.

Doing yoga exercises in a heated environment also has very soothing effects. According to studies, harmful toxins are released from the body in the process, thus leaving you cleaner and healthier.

Bikram Yoga is not advisable for individuals with cardio-vascular diseases, because performing exercises in a very warm environment may put excessive strain on the heart. In fact,some healthy people experience adverse effects from exercising in a heated environment. For this reason, *it is best to seek the advice of a doctor before starting this type of yoga.*

Ashtanga Yoga

Also known as "power yoga", the primary focus of Ashtanga Yoga is to develop stamina and strength through strong flowing movements. This is ideal for individuals who have successfully recovered from various back injuries. Athletic individuals are the ones who commonly practice AshtangaYoga.

Mantra Yoga

In Mantra Yoga the student uses potent sounds during meditation. Mental or verbal repetition of sounds like, "hum", "ram", "om", is applied to liberate the mind, body, and spirit.

Vini Yoga

In this yoga style, the individual learns how to effectively link movement and breathing into smooth and flowing exercises. Since the poses of Vini Yoga are very adaptable, people with neck or back problems can benefit greatly from it.

Bhakti yoga

Generally recognized as a devotional yoga, the primary focus of Bhakti yoga is the complete surrender of the self to the Divine.

Kundalini Yoga

Among all types of yoga, Kundalini Yoga is considered to be the most exceptional.

Its primary focus is on developing breathing techniques mixed with different yoga poses in order for an individual to reach a certain condition of enlightenment.

Because of its vaguely spiritual nature, you might be slightly put off as a beginner if your purpose for doing yoga is primarily to develop strength, fitness, and flexibility.

Raja Yoga

With the primary focus on meditation, the main objective of Raja Yoga is self-liberation. This type is only suitable for individuals who are capable of sustainable intense concentration..

Warm-Up Exercises

Great, we are ready to begin! As I mentioned ealier, it is important to beging each session with warm-up exercises.

These exercises make use of gentle poses that loosen and relax the body. They help expand the lungs, improve concentration, and warm the muscles, which lowers the risk of injury.

We will look at exercises such as

- Forward and back bends
- Seated forward bends
- Arm swings
- Hip and arm rotation
- Back twists
- And a few more

Each exercise comes with instructions on how to perform it, and where possible, there are pictures included to give you a better idea of what the exercise is all about.

Let's start with the Forward Bend exercise:

Forward Bend

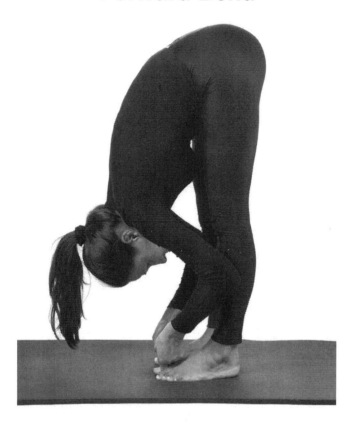

To perform the Forward Bend, begin with a wide stance with your feet pointed forward, keeping both your legs and knees straight.

Take a deep breath as you slowly stretch your back upward, extending both your arms above your head.

With your back still straight, carefully bend forward, pulling your head down through the legs. Touch the ground if you can.

Stay in this position for 10 seconds before releasing.

Back Bend

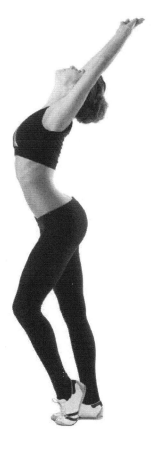

To do the Back Bend, start with your feet one meter apart, your feet pointed forward. You can place your hands either above your head, with your fingers pointed to the sky, or over your buttocks with your fingers pointed to the floor.

Pull your elbows and shoulders back to open chest. Slowly breathe in as you bend backward (as far as comfort allows).

Bend your knees to deepen the bend and to help you stay balanced. At this point, start breathing normally. Stay in this position for 10 seconds.

Release and slowly bring your body back to starting position.

Seated Forward Bend

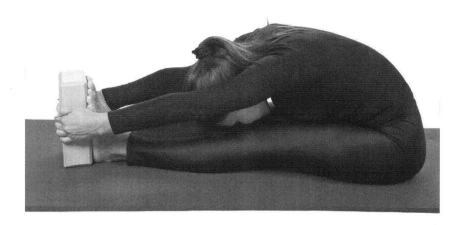

Begin the Seated Forward Bend by sitting straight.

Extend both legs forward. Keep them pressed together, knees straight.

Take deep breath. Breathe out slowly as you bend forward, placing both hands on each side of your legs. Slowly straighten up.

Repeat the process 10 times.

Back Twist

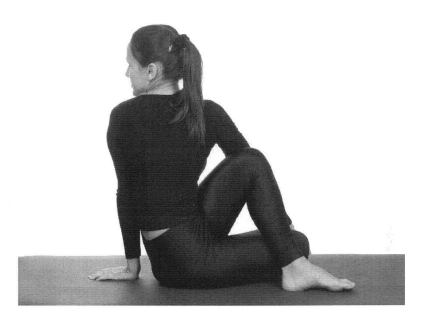

Start the Back Twist by sitting straight, your right leg forward, your left leg bent and crossed over the right leg.

Place your left palm flat on the ground.

Then slowly twist your body to the left as far out as you possibly can.

Hold this position for 10 seconds before repeating the process for your right side.

Repeat the sequence 10 times.

Butterfly

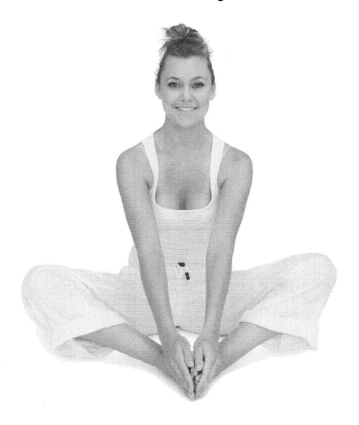

Begin the Butterfly position by sitting straight. Bend both legs with your soles touching each other close to the pelvis, imitating a butterfly.

While keeping your back straight, hold your toes with your hands as you roll your pelvis forward.

Move your knees in an upward and downward motion, your knees touching your arms as it moves upward.

Do this for 20 counts.

Then push your knees downward, slowly bending forward towards your feet while still keeping the back straight.

Try to touch your feet or the floor with your head. Repeat process 10 times.

Arm Rotation

To start the Arm Rotation exercise, begin with your feet one meter apart with your feet pointed forward.

Raise both your arms and spread them straight out from your body - shoulder level.

Create fists with your hands.

Create big circles (clockwise and counter clockwise) and with your arms keeping them straight.

Repeat the process 10 times.

Arm Swings

Begin Arm Swings by holding both your arms at shoulder level.

Slowly swing your arms forward and backward then cross them in the front and in the back.

Repeat this step 10 times.

Hip Rotation

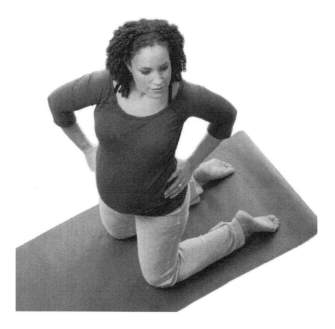

Start the Hip Rotation by placing both your hands on your hips.

You can either keep your legs straight or be in your knees.

Make big hip rotations as far out as you possibly can.

Do clockwise hip rotations 10 times then counter-clockwise 10 times.

Full Body Traction

To perform the Full Body Traction exercise, stand straight while keeping your feet together.

Interlock both your hands and raise your arms over your head with palms facing up.

Breathe in as you bring your arms closer to your ears.

Then while pulling your stomach in, rise on your tiptoes.

Hold this position to a count of 10.

Breathe out as you slowly return your heels back on the ground.

Repeat this process 10 times.

Breathing (Pranayama)

The breath wanders, the mind is unsteady, but when breath is stil, so is the mind still. – Hatha Yoga Pradipika

Now that we have reviewed some warm-up exercises to help you prepare your body for yoga, let's move on to another important aspect of the discipline – breathing, or in Sanskrit, Pranayama.

Pranayama is the science of breath control and is one of yoga's five basic principles. The term was derived from the words Prana which means life force, Yama which means control and Ayama which means expansion. Pranayama is not just about taking deep, healthy breaths. It is about opening the inner life force to prepare for meditation.

Normal breathing involves breathing in oxygen and breathing out carbon dioxide. The art of Pranayama aims to attain a balance between these two actions. Absorbing prana through controlled breathing will successfully link the mind, body, and spirit.

Pranayama consists of four stages:

- **Arambha** is the initial stage where one's interest in Pranayama is awakened.

- **Ghata** is the stage where the three sariras (causal, gross and subtle) envelopes the soul.

- **Parichay** is the stage where one experiences the Pranayama knowledge.

- **Nispatti** is the final stage where one goes beyond the physical body and meets with the Supreme.

The Benefits of Pranayama

1. Most of us unconsciously breathe from our chest, only using a fraction of our lungs. Shallow breathing can cause a variety of health problems. Through Pranayama, you will learn to breathe properly. This will help improve lung capacity, bringing a sufficient supply of oxygen to all parts of the body.

2. Breath control helps improve focus and concentration, which, in turn, alleviates anxiety and stress. As a result, you will achieve a clear, peaceful mind.

3. Pranayama aids in digestion. Learning how to breathe properly improves metabolism. It is also known to help release toxins from the body.

4. Through Pranayama, you will achieve a relaxed mind and body, leading to a successful spiritual journey.

Start Breathing Better Today!

Shallow breathing is a sign that you are experiencing stress. Correcting the way you breathe will help prevent many health problems; and, , prepare you for Pranayama, if your are a committed yogi.
Here's how you can start breathing better:

- **Be conscious about your posture.** A sunken chest and rounded shoulders deprive your lungs of oxygen intake. By improving your posture and opening your chest, you are giving your organs some breathing space.

- **Keep your stomach relaxed when breathing.** Most people squeeze their stomachs when told to take a deep breath. This restricts oxygen intake. A relaxed stomach enables your diaphragm and lungs to expand fully.

- **Breathe through your nose, not your mouth.** Nasal breathing always trumps breathing through the mouth. The nose filters the air we breathe in while the mouth bypasses this process. Also, since the nose is a smaller passageway, the air we inhale is breathed out more slowly, allowing the lungs to extract more oxygen from it.

A helpful tip: Lie down flat on the floor and place your right hand on top of your chest and your left one on top of your stomach. Take a deep breath and observe which hand rises higher. If your right hand rises higher, it means you are a chest breather and not utilizing your diaphragm properly.

Take the time to practice breathing techniques and exercises to help you breathe correctly. Pranayama is one of the most important elements of yoga and if not done right, it defeats the purpose of the whole discipline.

Breathing Warm-Up Exercises

Before practicing breathing techniques, it is important to do a few warm-ups first. Breathing warm-up exercises will energize you and quick-start your breathing.

Abdominal Breathing

Abdominal breathing is a relaxing exercise that will help you ultimately achieve mastery over your breathing. The method described in the following paragraph isolates and strengthens the abdominal breathing muscles. It also encourages fuller breathing and enhances awareness of your breaths.

To perform *Abdominal Breathing*, start by lying down on your back with your hands relaxed at your sides. Make sure that your neck, your spine, and your legs are aligned.

Then, take a deep breath in while pushing your belly out, then, squeeze your belly as you breathe out. Do this for 1-3 minutes, then do it again (faster this time) six times.

Finally, do another set (even faster this time) six times. If your chest remains still and only your belly is moving, it means that you are doing the exercise correctly.

Abdominal Lifts

The *Abdominal Lift* is another great warm-up for Pranayama exercises. It will help loosen and strengthen your abdominal breathing muscles as well as your lower back.

Start with a sitting position, your elbows wide open to enable your abdominals to move freely.

Without breathing in, breathe out all the way, squeezing out every last bit of air from your lungs. Then tuck your belly up as far as you can without breathing before dropping it back down. Do as many lifts as you can before your breath catches up to you. 3-5 lifts are ideal for beginners.

Butterfly Breathing

This warm-up exercise will wake up your breathing. It is also known to loosen the arms, neck, and shoulders while oxygenating the entire body.

To perform *Butterfly Breathing*, begin by standing straight, with your hands in prayer position in front of your chest.

Slightly tilt your pelvic area to protect your lower back during this exercise. Then, lace your fingers under your chin with your palms facing downward. Slowly raise your elbows upward while breathing in.

Next, lower your elbows as you breathe out, rolling your hands into a fist under your chin. Slowly push your chin up and back so that your neck stretches backward.

Do as many as you like.Start with 3-6 times.

Pranayama Techniques and Exercises for Beginners

Alternate Nostril Breathing (Nadi Sodhana)

The *Alternate Nostril Breathing* exercise will help balance your breathing while relaxing your body.

Start with a comfortable sitting position. Fold both your pointer and middle finger of your right hand into your palm. Only your thumb, ring, and pinky fingers should be left sticking up.

Next, bring your ring finger to the left side of your nose and your thumb to the right side.

Close your right nostril with your thumb before breathing in from your left nostril. Close your left nostril with your ring finger, open your right nostril and breathe out through it.

Continue alternating for 5-10 times.

Equal Breath (Sama Vritti Pranayama)

The *Equal Breath* breathing exercise aims to match the length of your inhale and exhale. It also helps enhance calmness and concentration.

Begin with a comfortable seated position. Close your eyes and observe your natural breath for about 30 seconds. Then, count to four slowly as you inhale, doing the same as you exhale. Continue this exercise for 5-10 minutes.

Three-Part Breath (Dirga Pranayama)

The *Three-Part Breath* aims to calm the entire body, keep the mind grounded, and increase awareness of the present moment.

Lie down on your back with your eyes closed, keeping the rest of your body loose and relaxed. Observe your natural breath for about 30 seconds. Then, breathe in deeply through your nose, filling your belly with air. As you exhale push your navel toward your spine to empty your belly of air. Do this deep belly breathing for 5 breaths.

Then, inhale deeply and fill your belly with air again; this time drawing a little more breath so that it expands to the rib cage, causing it to widen.

When you exhale, breathe air out from the rib cage first; then, push your navel back towards the spine to let all the air out. Repeat this step for 5 breaths.

To finish, repeat the inhale with the belly and the rib cage, this time drawing a little more air to fill the upper chest all the way up to the collar bone. When releasing the air, start with the chest; then the rib cage; and finally, the belly. Repeat this step for 5 times.

Cleaning Breath (Kalapabhati Pranayama)

The *Cleaning Breath* breathing exercise is known to help cleanse the body of toxins. This invigorating exercise also cleans the air inside the body.

Begin the *Cleaning Breath* with a cross-legged sitting position. Inhale and exhale deeply through the nose 2-3 times to prepare. Inhale comfortably; then, exhale sharply drawing your belly in.

Continue inhaling passively and exhaling forcefully for 30 breaths at a fast pace. End this exercise by inhaling and exhaling deeply through the nose 2-3 times.

If you feel lightheaded, go back to normal breathing.

Cooling Breath

This Pranayama *Cooling Breath* exercise helps cool the body. It is usually performed to finish an intense yoga session or used during hot weather.

Start with a comfortable cross-legged position. Take 2-3 deep inhales and exhales to prepare. Then roll your tongue, curling the sides towards the center. If you're having difficulty doing this, you can purse your lips to form a small letter O.

Next, inhale through the tube of your tongue or mouth, exhaling through the nostrils. Repeat this step 5-10 times or until you feel the cooling effect.

Yoga Exercises and Poses (Asanas)

Congratulations for making it this far! It is time to move on to the heart and soul of yoga – asanas.

There are six fundamental types of postures: backbends, balances, forward bends, inversions, standing poses and twists. However, there are thousands of variations, which means that you will always be learning something new in yoga. You will be awed by how many types of asanas the human body can perform.

With yoga, you will be able to reach places mentally and do things physically that you never thought possible.

If you are hesitant because of your flexibility (or lack thereof), you don't need to worry. I used to have the same concern.

Many years ago when I was just starting with the discipline, I wasn't exactly the most flexible person. I created a mantra of the 3 C's to motivate myself – Commitment, Consistency, and Change.

To be able to move forward with yoga, you have to have a steady anchor first - a commitment to the discipline.

Next, you have to be consistent. I don't recommend that you only practice whenever you feel like it or when you are in pain. Regular practice is vital to your success.

It s important to recognize your weaknesses and accept change within your mental, physical, and spiritual self. If you are not open to change, you will not be able to experience the great power that yoga offers you.

As a beginner, I recommend that you start learning from the bottom up. Mastering the most basic asanas will prepare your body for the more complicated ones. Remember, every yoga expert, including me, started from the bottom.

On the following pages you will find pictures and explanations of yoga exercises and poses for beginners to help you get started.

Standing Poses

Mountain Pose

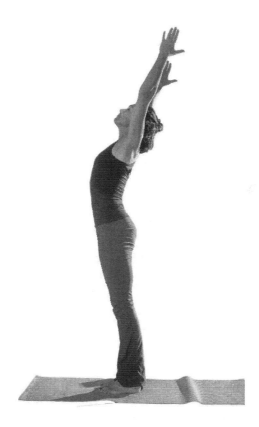

The *Mountain Pose*, also referred to as Tadasana, is the foundation of all yoga poses and the most basic standing position.

It helps develop your posture, strengthen your abdomen, ankles, buttocks, knees and thighs, provide relief against body tension and pain, and ease flat feet. The *Mountain*

Pose is also known to aid in digestion, to boost blood circulation, and to heighten body awareness.

Start by standing tall, keeping both feet together.

Relax your shoulders, evenly distributing weight through your arms, sides and, soles of your feet.

Inhale deeply.

Slowly raise hands overhead, with arms straight and your hands in prayer position. Reach upward as far as you can go.

For this posture to be effective make sure that your body is in perfect alignment. Keep your neck long, with your shoulder blades sliding down the back.

Also, draw in your belly slightly, widen your shoulders making sure they are parallel to your pelvis, and engage your quadriceps so that your knee caps will rise.

As a beginner you should do this pose with your back against the wall so that you can properly feel the alignment.

Downward Facing Dog

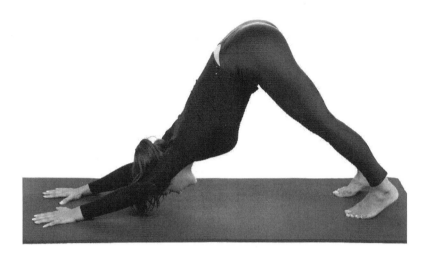

The *Downward Facing Dog* also referred to as Adho Mukha Svanasana, is a basic yoga pose for resting and strengthening the whole body.

It relieves back pain by releasing spine pressure; stretches and strengthens lower back and leg muscles; tones the arms, chest, hand, wrist, shoulder and upper back muscles; and promotes overall body circulation. It is also known to promote digestion and alleviate insomnia.

The *Downward Facing Dog* is usually executed many times in a yoga session. It is also one of the basic yoga postures that beginners need to learn.

Begin this pose by positioning yourself on all fours with your hands under your shoulders and your knees under your hips.

Curl your toes before pushing them back to raise your hips and straighten your legs.

Then, carefully move your hands forward a few inches, fingers spread wide.

Slowly raise your hips upward. Your body should form a reverse V.

Press your shoulders down, away from your ears and toward your hips.

Hold this position for 10 counts.

For beginners, practice by bending your arms and your knees slightly and by keeping your feet a few inches apart until you develop the skill to do the Downward Dog correctly.

Warrior Pose 1

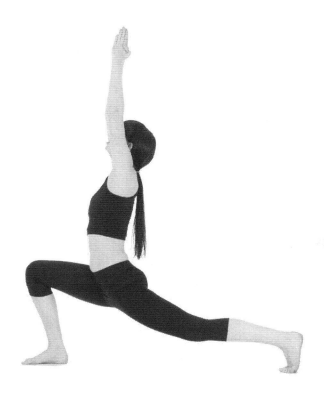

The *Warrior I* pose or Virabhadrasana is a standing yoga position that will help you learn how to be in the moment.

Some of its benefits include strengthening the ankles, back, legs and feet; increasing lung capacity; expanding the chest; enhancing stability; and improving flexibility of the hips.

Begin the *Warrior I* pose by standing straight with your legs spread 3-4 inches apart.

Turn the right foot to a 90-degree angle, left foot slightly turned in.

Next, bend your right knee directly over your right ankle, making sure that your thigh is parallel to the floor and your hips are square to the front.

Then, slowly raise both your arms, your palms facing each other, and your fingers apart.

Turn your head upward to gaze at your hands, sliding your shoulder blades down which will move you into a slight back bend position.

Triangle Pose

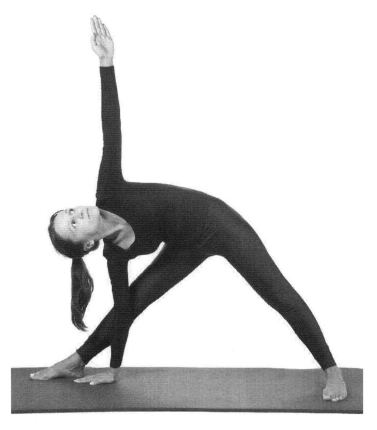

The Triangle Pose or Utthita Trikonasana is another basic yoga standing pose.

It helps build up and establish upper leg and lower back strength and releases tension from both areas. This pose will also help you develop balance and coordination; stretch your calves, groins, hamstrings, hips and spine; boost your digestion; and alleviate anxiety and stress.

Precision and concentration are needed to execute the Triangle Pose properly, Start the Triangle Pose by standing straight with your legs spread 3-4 feet apart.

Turn the left foot on a 45-degree angle and your right foot on a 90-degree angle.

Extend both arms out straight to your sides. Slowly bend to your right and touch the ground with your right hand. (Touch your knee if the ground is too difficult to reach.)

Stretch left arm toward the sky. Turn your face to look up at your left hand and hold the position for 10 slow counts. Slowly stand-up straight and repeat the process for the opposite side.

Beginners can practice the Triangle Pose by placing the right hand higher up on the leg if the floor is too difficult to reach at first. (Do not place it directly on the knee.) It is more important to keep the right leg straight than to place the hand on the floor.

Practice until you can reach the floor.

Seated Poses

Cobbler's Pose

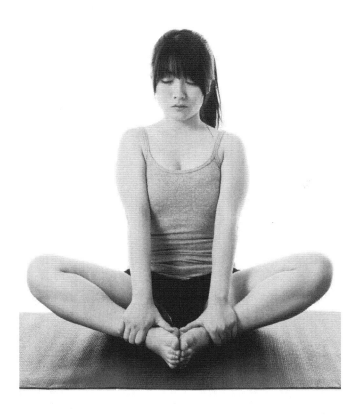

The Cobbler's Pose or sometimes referred to as the Bound Angle Pose is Badhha Konasana in Sanskrit. It is taught in every beginner yoga class.

The Cobbler's Pose opens the groin and the hips. It is also a position known to help relax the mind and prepare for meditation.

To do the Cobbler's Pose, begin with a comfortable cross-legged position.

While keeping your knees bent, bring the soles of your feet together which will force your knees to fall out to the sides.

Keep your spine long.

Then, wrap each hand around the corresponding foot. With your thumbs apply firm pressure to the outer edges of the feet.

Beginners can use blocks to support the knees. A padding mat can also be used to support the sit bones.

Easy Pose

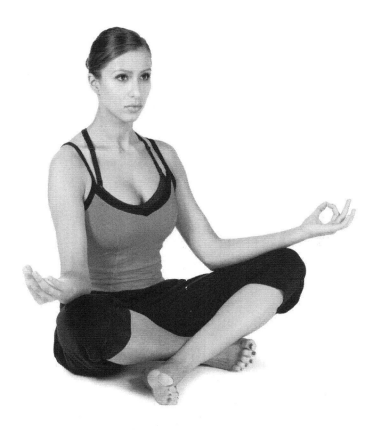

The Easy Pose, or Sukhasana in Sanskrit is basically a comfortable, cross-legged sitting position. As its name suggests, this type of asana is a good starting point for beginners. It is one of the most basic seated poses and is often used to begin breathing and meditation exercises.

Sukhasana is known to help calm the mind; stretch the ankle and knees; and strengthen the back.

Start with cross-legged seated position. Make sure that your spine is long, your shoulders are relaxed, and your chest is open.

Point one of your heels towards the groin.

The other foot may rest on the floor or may be rested on your lap.

Beginners can use padding under the sit bones to ensure that the hip bones will come above the knees. You can also opt to do this pose with your back against the wall to check your alignment.

Seated Forward Bend

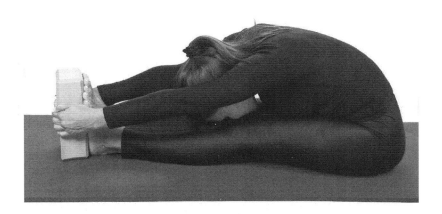

The Seated Forward Bend or Paschimottanasana is another basic yoga pose. It means 'intense stretch of the west' and is derived from the Sanskrit words pashima which means West and uttana which means intense stretch.

It is known for many benefits such as soothing headaches and menstrual discomforts; stretching the hamstrings, shoulders and spine; stimulating the kidneys; and stimulating the liver, ovaries and uterus.

It is also a good position to practice to relieve anxiety and stress.

Begin the Paschimottanasana with a seated position with your legs close together and stretched out in front of you.

Take a deep breath and make sure that your back is straight.

As you breathe out slowly bend your upper body forward toward your knees, hinging at the hips.

On each inhale, draw the spine long and on each exhale, bend a little farther.

Do this until you've reached as far as you can go. Then, hold your ankles for support.

Stay in this position for 1-3 minutes.

Beginners are advised to use padding under the sit bones for support. You can also take hold of your shins while you are bent over if the ankles are too difficult to reach at first.

Staff Pose

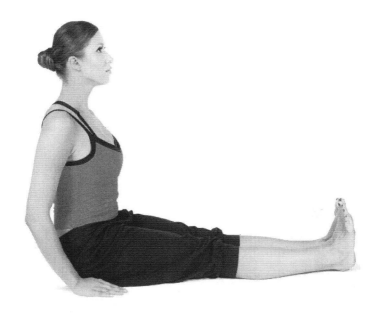

The Staff Pose, also referred to as Dandasana is where all other yoga seated positions originated. Many experts note it to be the seated version of the Mountain Pose (Tadasana).

The Staff Pose helps improve alignment; stretches the chest and the shoulders; and strengthens the back muscles.

Begin the Staff Pose by sitting comfortably on the floor with your legs outstretched in front of your torso.

Engage your thigh muscles and make your spine long.

Relax your arms at both sides and place your hands on the floor palm down.

Straighten your shoulders and make sure they directly above your hips.

Stay in this position for 1 minute or longer.

If you are a beginner, you can use padding under your sit bones or opt to do this position with your back against the wall.

Pigeon Pose

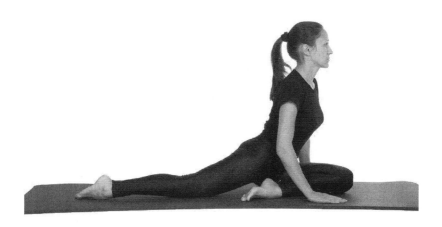

Pigeon Pose, also referred to as EkaPadaRajakapotasana, is a hip-opener pose.

Studies show that tightness in the hips is a result of built up tension and stress.

Doing the Pigeon Pose could enhance hip flexibility. This pose is also very good for stretching various deep glutes, Stretching your groins and enhancing stimulation of the internal organs. If you are suffering from sciatic pain or urinary disorders, this pose will help you eliminate those as well.

Start the pose with a push-up position, aligning your palms with the shoulders.

Position the left knee near the shoulder and your left heel close to the right hip.

Lift your chest up while keeping your upper body straight.

Breathe slowly for one minute. Then switch sides.

Repeat the process 5 times.

Supine Poses

Child's Pose

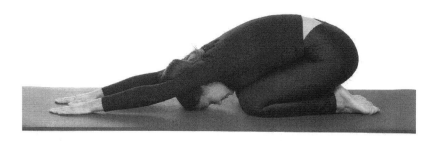

The *Child's Pose* or Balasana is derived from the Sanskrit word *bala* which translates to child in English.

It is a basic yoga resting/supine pose which calms the mind and alleviates stress. It also gently stretches the ankles, hips and thighs and effectively relieves back and neck pain.

The Balasana is an important pose that beginners need to learn. It can be used as a resting position when one gets tired or out of breath. It is one of the most common relaxation poses in yoga.

Start the *Child's Pose* with a kneeling position with your big toes together.

Sit on your heels and separate your knees just enough for your torso to fit through between them.

You can also opt to spread your knees as wide as the mat, whichever is easier for you. Keep your toes together.

Then, slowly bend forward, bringing your belly to rest between your thighs and your forehead to the floor.

Your arms can either be stretched out in front of you with palms facing downward or at the back alongside the thighs with your palms facing upward, as shown in the picture below.

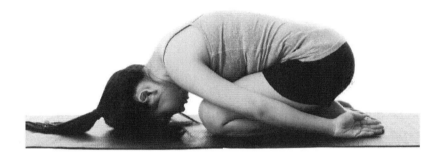

Stay in this position for 30 seconds to a few minutes.

Corpse Pose

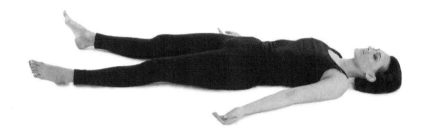

The Corpse Pose, or Savasana in Sanskrit, was derived from the term sava which means corpse. It is also sometimes referred to as Mrtasana.

This pose is used to symbolically "die" along with our habits and enter into a dimension of neutrality.

It is often used to end an asanas routine and help the body "breathe" and rest.

To do the Corpse Pose, start by lying comfortably on the floor. Make sure that your body is aligned and evenly resting on the floor.

Bring your arms alongside your body with your palms facing up. Allow your feet to fall out at either side.

Take a deep breath. As you exhale, relax your whole body from your bones to your muscles.

Then, calm your senses and clear your mind. Focusing on your breathing might help.

Lastly, let go of everything – imagine your body melting onto the floor. Release any tension and let your body feel heavy.

Stay in this position for 5 minutes for every 30 minutes of asanas routine.

.

Legs up the Wall

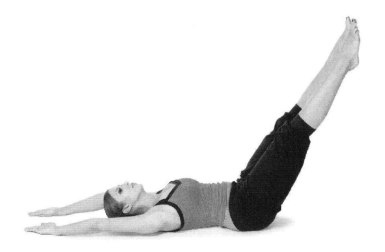

The Legs up the Wall Pose is also known as Viparita Karani, derived from the Sanskrit words viparita which means reversed and karani which means action.

This is the pose to practice if you have cramped feet and tired legs at the end of the day. It helps soothe back ache and stretches the front torso as well as the back of the neck and legs.

The Viparita Karani is also used to calm the mind.

Start this position by sitting with your side next to a wall and your knees bent into the chest.

Then, slowly lean backward while bringing your legs up into the wall. Use your elbows for support.

Once your legs are comfortable on the wall, release the elbows and lie down on your back. Relax both arms at each side.

Stay in this pose anywhere from 5-15 minutes.

To come out of this position, simply bring your knees to your chest and roll to your side.

As a beginner, it is recommended that you use a bolster or thick, folded blankets to support your spine. If you are stiff, place the support farther from the wall. If you are flexible, place the support closer to the wall.

Supine Spinal Twist

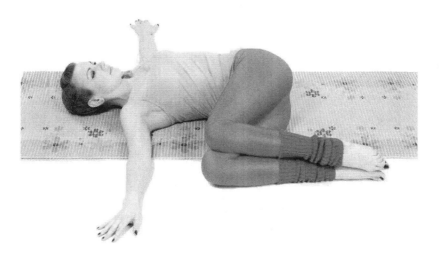

The Supine Spinal Twist or Supta Matyendrasana is another yoga resting position.

Like any twist position, the Supta Matyendrasana is known for its balancing and toning powers. It also helps improve breathing, poor digestion, low energy, and a variety of body aches and pains. It also stretches the glutes, and relaxes the spine.

To perform the Supine Spinal Twist, begin by lying comfortably on the ground.

Bend your knees so that the soles of your feet are against the floor.

Lift your hips slowly and shift them about an inch to your right.

Stretch your left leg on the floor.

Then, bring your right knee to your chest before dropping it over to the left side of your body.

Extend your hands at both sides in a straight line with the palms facing down.

Slowly turn your head to the right.

Hold this position for 5-10 breaths.

Slowly bring your right knee back into your chest before repeating the steps for the other side.

Backbend Poses

Cobra Pose

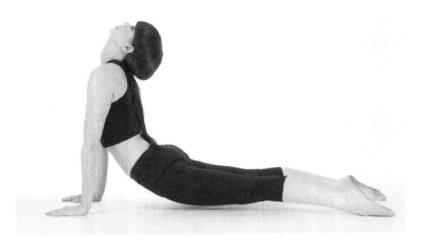

The *Cobra Pose*, also known as Bhujangasana is highly recommended for individuals who constantly suffer from lower back pain. It is usually done as part of the Sun Salutation Vinyasa sequence.

The Bhunjanasana offers plenty of benefits such as strengthening the arms, spine and shoulders; alleviating menstrual irregularities; anxiety and stress; promoting healthy blood circulation; and clearing the heart and lung passages by opening the chest.

Begin the *Cobra Pose* by lying on the mat face down.

Place your palms under shoulders and extend both your legs with the tops of your feet touching the ground.

Slowly raise your upper body upward with your palms supporting the weight.

Engaging your legs and pressing them down will help you lift your chest higher.

Raise your face toward the sky.

Stay in position for a minute. Relax and repeat the process 5 times.

Bridge Pose

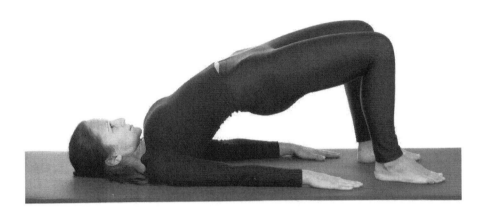

The Bridge Pose, also referred to as Half Wheel is Setu Bandhasana in Sanskrit. This position promotes stress reduction and relaxation.

In this pose, the hips and legs mainly do the work, which in turn alleviates tired feet.

Other benefits of the Bridge Pose include strengthening the spine; improving the flexibility of the spine; enhancing blood circulation; boosting digestion; and relieving symptoms of asthma and high-blood pressure.

Start the Bridge Pose by lying flat on the floor.

Bend your knees directly over the heels and position your arms on your sides with the palms facing down.

Slowly lift your hips, Make sure that your thighs are parallel to the floor.

Press your feet firmly on the ground. Your hands must be clasped under your lower back with your arms pressed down.

Then, bring your chest close to your chin. Hold this position for a minute.

You can also place pillows underneath for easier execution.

Cow Pose

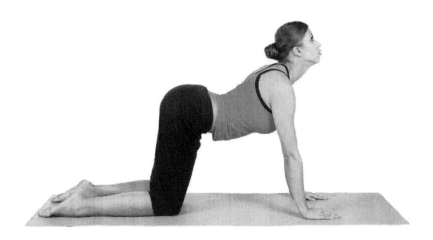

The Cow Pose or Bitilasana is another basic yoga back bend position.

It is known to be a stress-fighter. It provides a gentle massage to the belly organs as well as the spine. It also stretches the neck and front of the torso.

The Legs up the Wall Pose or Viparita Karani is a good preparatory pose for the Cow Pose.

Start the Legs up the Wall Pose with your hands and knees on the floor, forming a tabletop position.

Make sure that your knees are directly below your hips and that both your elbows and shoulders are perpendicular to the floor.

Take a deep breath.

Then, slowly lift your chest and sitting bones upwards which will cause your belly to sink downwards.

Also lift your head and look forward.

Next, exhale and slowly return to the tabletop position.

Repeat the steps 10-20 times.

Balancing Poses

Tree Pose

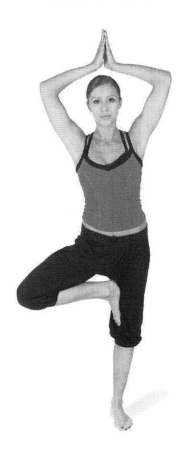

The Tree Pose or Vrksasana is one of the most basic yoga balancing poses.

It is done to improve balance; strengthen the ankles, back, calves and thighs; enhance concentration; and improve concentration.

Constant practice will also improve groin and hip flexibility. The Tree Pose is ideal for individuals with flat feet or sciatica.

Begin the Vrksasana by standing straight with both arms placed on the sides.

Slowly shift your weight with only the left leg as support.

Carefully position the sole of your right foot just inside your left thigh.

Find your balance.

Palms together, bring both hands in front of your chest similar to a prayer position.

Slowly raise your arms towards the sky with your palms still stuck together.

Stay in position for 30 seconds to a minute. Slowly lower right leg before repeating the process for the left leg.

Plank Pose

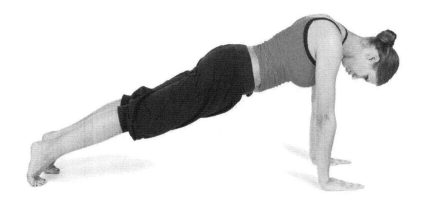

The Plank Pose is usually done after doing the Downward Facing Dog Pose (Adho Mukha Svanasana).

It is a basic balancing pose that is used to strengthen the arms, wrist and spine and to tone the abdominal muscles.

The Plank Pose is also used as preparation for more complicated arm balancing poses.

To perform the Plank Pose, start from the Downward Facing Dog position.

From there, bring your torso forward until your whole body is in a straight line and your shoulders are directly above your wrists.

Imagine that you are about to do a push-up to get the position right.

Then, press your hands and forearms down to the floor and press back through your heels.

Broaden your shoulder blades and make sure that your chest doesn't sink.

Stay in this position for 10 slow counts.

Warrior III Pose

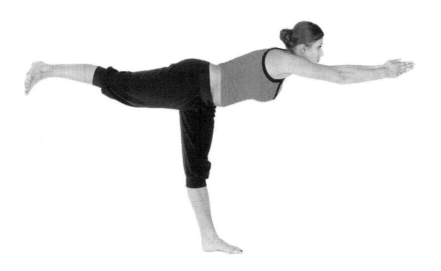

Also called the Virabhadrasana III, the Warrior III Pose is a combination of backward and forward bending elements. It is one of the more challenging yoga beginner poses but can be easily mastered through practice and patience.

The Warrior III Pose helps strengthen the ankles, the back, the legs and the shoulders. It is also known to help tone the whole body and to improve posture. Lastly, it helps sharpen focus and concentration.

To practice Virabhadrasana III, start in Tadasana (Mountain Pose) position.

Carefully extend your right foot forward about 12 inches, focusing your weight onto your right leg.

Take a deep breath as you raise your arms over your head in prayer position.

As you exhale, slowly lift your left leg up. Follow through by lowering your upper body towards the floor to help keep your balance.

Your right leg should be perpendicular to the floor and your body parallel to the floor. Keep your arms outstretched above your head.

Stay in this position anywhere from 30 seconds to 1 minute.

Beginners can start practicing the Warrior III pose with a partner or against the wall to help keep balance.

Crow Pose

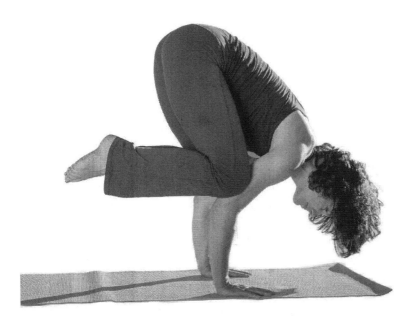

The Crow Pose or Bakasana is one of the more complicated yoga balancing poses for beginners. It is also referred to as the Crane Pose. Bakasana is derived from the Sanskrit word baka which means crane.

This position stretches the entire length of the back. In the process, the arms, shoulders and joints are strengthened as well, developing your sense of concentration, balance, and coordination in the process.

Start from the Downward Facing Dog Pose (Adho Mukha Svanasana); bend your elbows and slowly lift your heels from the floor.

Rest your knees against your outer arm. Keep your toes on the floor with your abs firmly engaged.

Then, press your legs against your arms.

Hold this position for 10 breaths.

Relaxation and Meditation

Congratulations, new yogis! I am very proud that you've come this far. Now, it's time for us to discuss yet another vital part of yoga – meditation.

In yoga, there is a fundamental unity called *advaita* which is a unique methodology that exists within the discipline's tradition. This union is designed to reveal every living thing's interconnectedness. Meditation is the actual experience of *advaita.*

According to the Yoga Sutra, this union takes place only when the mind is clear and quiet. Patanjali, the one who compiled the verses in the Yoga Sutra says that once you accept that your non-stop cravings for pleasure and material things that can never be satisfied, meditation begins. When your external quest turns inward, it means that you are already in the realm of meditation.

In the dictionary, the word meditation simply means to ponder upon or to contemplate. In the yogic context, however, meditation or *dhyana* is known to be the state of pure consciousness.

In Patanjali's eight-limbed system, Dhyana is the seventh limb/stage, following *dharana* (concentration) and followed by *samadhi* (enlightenment or self-realization).

When we concentrate, we usually focus on one object that is apart from ourselves. However, if we want to go into meditation, we must get involved with this object. Communicating with the object will bring us into a deep awareness that there is no difference between the object and ourselves. This will, in turn, bring us to *samadhi.*

Think of it as establishing a new relationship. Concentration is like meeting someone new and making contact with that person.

Meditation, on the other hand is getting to know that person – spending time together, sharing, and listening to stories, etc. Eventually you and that person will develop a deep friendship, partnership or marriage. You and that person become one.

Before starting with meditation, there are a few important things that you must consider:

Time and Place

The time and place for meditation is are two of the most important factors in the whole process. It is important to meditate at the same time and in the same place every day for consistency.

Choose a quiet, well-ventilated place in your home where you will not be disturbed.

Personally, I think that the optimal time for a meditation is during the morning when your mind is still clear and you can't be distracted from the demands of the day. However, if you do not have time in the morning, meditate in the late afternoon or early evening.

For beginners, 5-10 minutes of meditation should suffice when it is being done after asanas in a yoga class. If you are meditating independently at home, a 15 to 20-minute time frame is usually manageable when you are first starting.

Posture

Choose a position that is comfortable for you. After all, being uncomfortable defeats the purpose of the whole process. If you choose to sit (on a chair or on the floor), keep your spine long and the rest of the body relaxed. Rest your hands comfortably on your thighs either palms up or down.

If you prefer standing or walking, it is still important to keep your spine long and to relax the rest of the body. Your arms should hang freely and comfortably at your sides.

If you prefer to meditate in a supine position, keep your body in a comfortable, symmetrical position. Use support for your head and/or knees, if necessary.

Preparation

It is ideal to take a quick shower before meditation. Even a splash of water on your face will help you feel refreshed. Make sure that you also empty your bladder as well as the bowels to prevent distractions during meditation.

Do not try to meditate immediately after eating. You should allow several hours to pass after a meal before you meditate. But, if it has been a long day and you must eat, take only a light snack and allow at least half an hour before starting to meditate.

How to Begin Meditation

Now that you are ready to begin meditation, follow these simple steps:

1. Do some light stretches.

Before getting into your preferred meditation position, take a few minutes to do some stretching.

Focus on your neck and spine – bending them forward, backward, and sideways.

2. Reflect.

Once you are comfortably in your meditation position, allow a few minutes for your mind to wander and reflect.

Think about your daily activities, your life in general, or your spiritual purpose.

This will allow the mind to naturally settle down.

3. Be aware of your body.

Close your eyes at this point, allowing yourself to explore your body - part by part using your inner attention. Increasing your awareness of your body will further help you focus.

4. Focus on your breath.

Keeping your eyes closed, shift your attention to the rhythm of your breathing.

Breath awareness is considered to be the most important focal point for beginning meditation. The easiest way to do this is to focus on the air as it flows through your nostrils. Feel the air come in and feel it go out.

5. Witness the flow of your thoughts.

Once you are in the meditative state, it is good to let your thoughts flow even when your mind is focused. Imagine that you are driving a car and your eyes are on the road, but your awareness is still absorbing everything else that is happening around you.

6. End your meditation by reversing the process.

It is ideal to come out of your meditative state the same way you came in. After meditation, briefly come back to breath awareness, then shift your focus to the entirety of your body before opening your eyes.

Benefits of Meditation in Everyday Life

According to research, both psychological and physiological changes in the body occur during meditation and deep relaxation. This, in turn, causes an actual shift in the brain function and in other body processes.

You know that taking some time off from work or school to relax provides mental and physical benefits. Now, imagine what deep relaxation can do for your mind and body.

Meditation helps in a variety of ways: body awareness, self awareness, attention regulation, and emotion regulation. Not only that, deep relaxation also provides a plethora of health benefits. Some are listed below.

Relieves Anxiety and Stress

Having the ability to control your thoughts and to clear your mind is the ultimate stress buster. According to the *Health Psychology Journal*, meditation not only relieves and prevents stress, but it is also linked to the decrease of cortisol, a stress hormone, in the body.

Increases Immunity

A study done at *Ohio State University* found that deep relaxation and meditation boosts the immunity of recovering cancer patients. According to the study, the daily practice of progressive muscular relaxation decreased the recurrence of breast cancer. Relaxation exercises also proved to kill cancer cells in the elderly, boosting their resistance against tumors and viruses.

Fights Against Mental Illness

A meditation technique called *Integrative Body-Mind Training* was found to cause some changes in the brain that may prevent or combat mental illnesses.

Researchers from the *University of Oregon* linked the practice of meditation to axonal density (increased signaling connections in the brain) and to the increased production of myelin, a protective tissue found in the brain.

Helps You Sleep Better

Meditation not only control moods and emotions, but it can also help provide a good night's sleep.

According to a study done at the *University of Utah*, people who regularly meditate have better control over their behaviors and emotions during the day. These people also experience less activation during bedtime which benefits them with a more quality sleep and even the ability to better manage stress in the future.

Increases Fertility

Stress has a negative impact on fertility. A study conducted at the *University of Western Australia* found that women are more likely to conceive when they are relaxed rather than stressed.

Furthermore, research at *Trakya University* in Turkey showed that stress lowers sperm count and motility and suggests that de-stressing by means of deep relaxation or meditation can boost both male and female fertility.

Aids in Weight Loss

The *American Psychological Association and Consumer Reports* conducted a survey among psychologists regarding the best strategies for weight loss. Seven out of 10 pyschologists in the survey consider meditation to be an excellent weight-loss strategy.

Allows YOU to Know Your True Self

Meditation can help you to discover the truth about yourself. It allows you to objectively analyze yourself.

According to a study done by the *Psychological Science Journal*, mindfulness will help you determine and overcome the blind spots that will either improve or worsen your flaws beyond reality.

Common Meditation Techniques

Just as there are many variations of asanas, there are also a variety of ways to meditate. The effectiveness of a method depends on the person's preference and level of comfort.

Common meditation techniques you can try as a beginner:

Using Sound

The first stage of meditation is to establish a point of focus. Many yogis find it easier to get into the meditative state by using sound as a point of focus.

Mantra Yoga (derived from the words *man* which means to think and *tra* which means instrumentality) employs the use of an affirmation, a phrase, or a sound as a focal point.

If you choose to go with an affirmation or a phrase, you have to state it out loud and repetitively with purpose and feeling as you start your meditation. A *Mantra Meditation* requires conscious engagement from the meditator.

As a beginner, you can start with affirmations such as, *I am calm and relaxed*; or *I am ready and alert*.

Using Imagery

Using imagery as a focal point is a common practice for beginners. Visualizing is a good way of helping you get into the zone.

In traditional yoga, the meditator uses the image of his/her chosen god/goddess to meditate. Other yogis meditate on the *chakras* (energy centers), focusing on the area of the body that corresponds to a particular chakra.

The easiest way to use imagery as your focal point is to visualize your favorite spot in nature. When I was a beginner, I used to imagine myself on a picturesque beach – the palm trees swaying in the gentle breeze, my feet buried in warm sand, and the golden rays of the sun touching my shoulders.

Gazing

Gazing is a variation of imagery. With this technique, you are required to choose an object in the room as your focal point for your meditation and maintain an open-eyed focus on it.

In yogic terms, gazing is referred to as *drishti* which means to view or gaze. It could be a painting on your wall, a flower on a vase or a candle.

A variety of Hatha Yoga asanas use gazing points. Drishti is especially emphasized in Hatha Yoga's Ashtanga. Many Pranayama techniques also require specific positioning of the eyes such as gazing at the *third eye.*

Breathing

Using your breathing as a point of focus is another meditation technique common to beginners. As in Pranayama practice, you count your breaths and observe everything, including every sensation – the temperature of your breath, the way it moves in your abdomen and torso, how it feels as it goes in and out, etc.

Breath observance is a Buddhist practice and is commonly used by practitioners of *vipassana* or Mindfulness Meditation. The Sanskrit word *vipassana* means to look deeply.

Physical Sensations

Observing a physical sensation is a meditation technique similar to breath observance. You focus on a particular sensation that draws your attention. This technique requires the same amount of detailed observations as you would use for observing your breath.

The easiest way is to choose and engage in a physical feeling that you currently have. It may be as simple as concentrating on how cold or hot your hands are feeling or something deeper like the strength of your spine.

This method is somewhat more complicated than breath observance but it will enhance focus and concentration during meditation practice for a beginner.

Meditation Exercises for Beginners

Now that you are more familiar with meditation techniques, you are ready to try some of the easier basic exercises that will help you prepare for more complicated ones in the future.

These exercises are excellent for building self-confidence, reducing stress, and for maintaining your general health and well-being.

Walking Meditation

This meditation exercise is good for calming the mind and increasing body awareness. It is common among monks in monasteries, which we all know are experts on the practice.

To begin the *Walking Meditation*, choose a quiet set path, preferably one that is circular or square. A garden or a sports field is ideal. Familiarize yourself with the path by walking through it a couple of times.

Once you are ready, go the beginning of the path and take a deep breath. Shift your focus to your body – be conscious about it and sense it. Then, breathe out as you start walking slowly.

While you are walking, notice how your body is functioning part by part. If a thought interferes with your concentration, try to push it away. Do this for 10-15 minutes.

Eating Meditation

The Eating Meditation is designed to increase your awareness of your unconscious eating habits as well as your body's hunger and fullness signals. It includes focusing on the different sensations of eating such as smelling, tasting, chewing, and swallowing. This exercise, when practiced regularly, will help you adopt a whole new approach to eating and relaxing.

For this meditation exercise, you will need a small piece of food such as a small piece of fruit or a cracker. Take a deep breath and relax your mind.

Explore your food by smelling it. Think about how this smell makes you feel or what comes to mind with this particular smell.

Then, shift your focus on the actual sensory experience of tasting and chewing. Do the same when you swallow the food. Observe the changes of the flavor's intensity in each moment. Take another bite and follow the same instructions.

Forgiveness Meditation

This healing meditation exercise will help you overcome negative experiences from your past. It is created to free oneself from negative emotions such as hatred, guilt, and regret and to embrace forgiveness and letting go.

For this exercise, choose an issue in your life that made you feel angry or disappointed – a simple one is best when you are doing this for the first time For example, you could choose a petty argument that you had this morning with your mother, friend, or spouse.

Begin to replay that experience in your mind and remember the conversation in as much detail as possible.

When you finish, replay the scenario again; but, this time focus only on your side of the conversation. Determine the things you said that may have hurt or offended the other person. Then, prepare an apology and imagine placing it in a pretty box and delivering the package to the person.

Next, take a deep breath before replaying the other side of the conversation. Listen carefully and think about what the other person is trying to point out.Try to put yourself in his/her shoes and how you would convey the same point.

Finally, think of an ideal, alternate scenario to what you actually experienced. Accept this in your heart as reality.

Inhale and exhale for 1-2 minutes. If you use affirmations for your meditation use them for this last step.

Recommended Exercise Sequence for Beginners

I believe that hard work deserves a reward. So, because you took the time and the effort to share your first yoga experience with me, I want to share with you the first yoga exercise sequence I learned and mastered when I was a beginner.

This sequence is designed to stretch the back, the hips and the hamstrings which are common problem areas for a lot of people.

Duration: 10-15 minutes

What you'll need: A yoga mat

Step 1: Allow a few minutes to calm the mind and to relax the body.

Step 2: When you are ready, lie on your back and perform Pelvic Tilts 20 times.

How to do Pelvic Tilts:

In supine position, bend your knees so that the soles of your feet are on the floor.

Your arms should be relaxed at both sides with your palms face down.

Then, without your butt leaving the floor, start rocking your hips gently towards your face.

You should be able to feel your lower back pressing against the floor.

Step 3: Continue to warm up your back by doing 10-15 Cat-Cow Stretches (Chakravakasana)

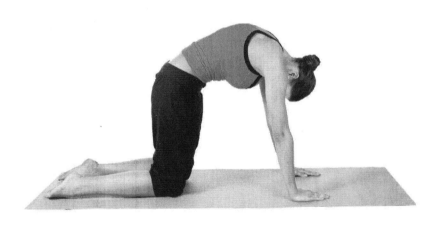

How to do the Cat-Cow Stretch:

The Cat-Cow Stretch involves transitioning between the Cow Pose and the Cat Pose.

From the Cow Pose, shift into the Cat Pose by dropping your head, rounding up the spine and releasing the tops of your feet onto the floor.

Step 4:

From the Cat-Cow Stretch, press back to the Downward Facing Dog Pose (Adho Mukha Svanasana) by pedalling your legs and bending your knees one after the other to reach each heel towards the floor.

Hold this pose for 10-15 breaths.

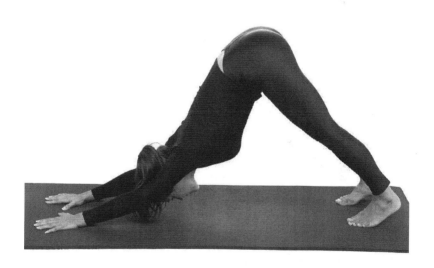

Step 5:

From the Downward Facing Dog Pose, walk your feet toward your hands until you are in a Standing Forward Bend (Uttanasana) position.

Stay for 10 breaths. If this is too difficult for you the first few times, come to a flat back with your hands on your shins or your fingertips on the floor.

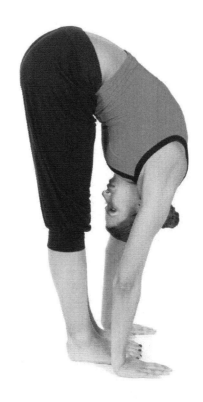

Step 6:

Then, slightly bend your knees and stand up to do the Mountain Pose (Tadasana).

Then, extend your arms at both sides before bringing them up toward the ceiling in prayer position which brings you to the Raised Arms Pose (Urdhva Hastasa).

Stay in this position for 10 breaths.

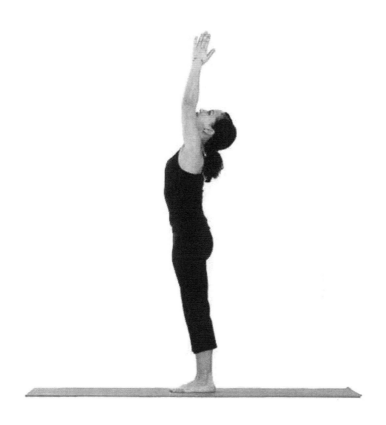

Step 7:

Using your right leg, take a big step forward and bend your right knee.

Extend your left leg at the back to transition to the Warrior 1 Pose (Virabhadrasana I). Hold this position for 10-15 breaths.

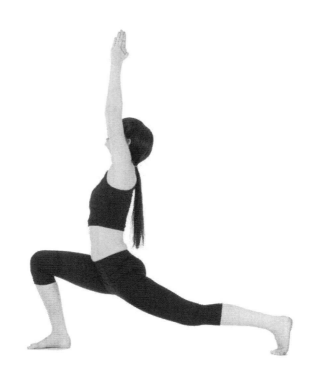

Step 8:

End your routine by spending a few minutes to rest in the Corpse Pose (Savasana).

This will allow your body to absorb the benefits of the routine you just performed.

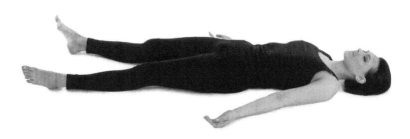

How to do the Corpse Pose:

Lie down on your back. Relax your entire body including the face.

Bring your arms alongside the body, slightly separated with the palms facing upwards.

Allow your feet to fall out to either side. Let your body become heavy.

Top Ten Yoga Tips

Whew! You've come a long way and I just want to say that I am so proud of you! I salute you for choosing to practice yoga for your mind, body, and spirit's health. And... I salute you all the more for learning it on your own.

While attending a yoga class may prove to be helpful in learning the discipline, practicing yoga in the comfort of your own home will make the experience more personal. After all, yoga is about achieving what YOU need.

With yoga you don't need special abilities to achieve your goals. All you need is the hunger to learn with the commitment to pursue the practice and you are good to go.

Remember, to be successful at anything, it is important to know only two things: the ground rules for the arena in which you are playing and yourself.

Top Ten Tips for a Fulfilling Yoga Workout

1. Create a sanctuary at home.

Choose a quiet spot in your home and dedicate it to your yoga practice. A clean, well-ventilated and serene place is ideal. Make sure you have ample space to perform various yoga asanas.

Decorating your sanctuary with images and objects that create peace in your heart will contribute to the success of your workouts.

2. Invest in the tools of the trade.

Learning anything new is easier if you have the proper tools. A yoga mat, a yoga blanket, a strap, two blocks, two bolsters and a zafu (meditation cushion) are your basic material needs when it comes to yoga.

There are variations of these tools to fit every budget and personal taste. I am sure you'll find some to your liking.

3. Learn all you can about yoga.

Research and seek advice from experienced yogis you may know. This is very important for beginners.

Knowing exactly what to do and what you are doing will lead to a more successful yoga workout.

4. Prevent injury.

Even if you think you are doing a yoga posture right on the first try, chances are there is still room for improvement. Never force a posture – if a part of your body hurts when in a posture or if you feel like you're going to tip over from a balancing pose, stop. Also, it is best to clear your yoga space of furniture and other obstacles for your safety.

Make sure to remove any carpets as well, if possible. Soft surfaces make balancing difficult and you could injure your joints.

Remember, an act of prevention is better than having to take care of an injury .

5. Make your yoga time a sacred time.

Inform everyone in your home that this particular hour or two is the time of your yoga workout. Explain that it is important that you not be interrupted.

Also, do not bring anything into your sanctuary that may distract you while practicing - mobile phones and tablets. Dedicate this time entirely to yourself and yoga.

6. Relax.

Take a quick shower to help you feel refreshed and more relaxed before your yoga workout especially if it is in the evening. This will also help clear your mind.

7. Set the mood.

You will not feel fulfilled at the end of your workout if you weren't feeling up to it in the beginning. Relax for a few minutes by listening to some relaxing yoga music.

8. Be patient.

Don't expect to do everything right the first few times; and don't be anxious about your progress. This will only lead to loss of focus during workouts. Just do your best to learn at your own pace. Give yourself some time to adjust to the practice.

9. Vary your routine periodically.

Once you are familiar with a routine, try a new one, and another new one after that to avoid boredom. Once your initial enthusiasm about yoga is gone, it's easy to get bored and simply quit.

10. Meditate.

The components of a fulfilling yoga workout are a relaxed body and a relaxed mind. After performing a series of asanas, make it a habit to do some meditation techniques to achieve peace of mind.

Top Ten Reasons for Practicing Yoga

In my introduction, I briefly discussed _why you **should** practice yoga_; but, you are the only one who can decide _why you **want to** practice yoga_. It is about your personal reasons and your personal needs.

For your consideration, I have listed below the top 10 reasons why people choose to get into yoga:

1. **For a healthier body.** The truth is, it us hard to maintain health given the environment we live in today. So, if you're looking for a new activity or hobby, you might as well choose something that will benefit your body and your health.

2. **For a healthier mind.** With your daily obligations and responsibilities, it's pretty normal to feel that your head is going to explode at any moment. Give your mind some peace by practicing the relaxing discipline of yoga.

3. **For weight loss.** Because fasting and weight loss diets are the craze right now, yoga is a healthy alternative to help maintain a healthy weight.

4. **For stress relief.** Nothing compares to clearing your mind and having the ability to control your thoughts. Yoga is simply the ultimate stress-buster.

5. **For discipline.** All the yoga asanas as well as the various breathing and meditation techniques

require mindfulness, patience, and practice – all helpful in learning the value of discipline and hard work.

6. **For better body awareness.** Yoga will help you know your body better and determine what it needs to function optimally.

7. **For self-growth.** Yoga is for EVERYONE. Whether you're flexible or not; as long as you're committed, you will definitely grow and progress.

8. **For a spiritual awakening.** No matter what this means to you or what you believe in, yoga will help you connect with your spiritual self.

9. **For a better perspective.** Yoga will help you see the world differently – the way you are, the way the world works, your relationship with people, and the things surrounding you.

10. **For a better YOU.** Through yoga you will learn to accept your flaws and improve them; build on your strengths; and get to know yourself and your body better.

Top Ten Benefits of Yoga

This is a quick review of the wonderful benefits that are in store for you when you practice yoga:

1. **Fights against anxiety and stress.** Yoga relaxes the body and lowers the levels of the stress hormone, cortisol.

2. **Reduces body aches and pains.** According to medical studies, practicing yoga poses, meditation, or the two combined help decrease pain for people suffering with arthritis, chronic back and neck pain, multiple sclerosis, hypertension and even cancer.

3. **Improves breathing.** Yoga's breathing techniques or Pranayama trigger the body's relaxation response, helps improve breathing, and helps increase lung capacity.

4. **Increases body strength.** Aside from relieving muscular tension, yoga stretches and strengthens all 600 muscles of the body, improving your strength from head to toe!

5. **Enhances flexibility**. Performing various yoga postures and exercises will help improve your flexibility, mobility, and range of motion – all of which are beneficial to decreasing the risk of injury.

6. **Improves circulation**. Through the different asanas and pranayama techniques, circulation is

improved and oxygenated blood moves more efficiently throughout the body.

7. **Improves body alignment**. Regular practice of yoga postures will help improve alignment over time. It will also relieve neck, back, joint, and muscle aches.

8. **Conditions the cardiovascular system**. Yoga has plenty of cardiovascular benefits including lowering resting heart rate, increasing oxygen uptake, and improving stamina while exercising.

9. **Sharpens focus and concentration.** Meditation techniques will help clear the mind and encourages proper focus and concentration.

10. **Provides an overall sense of well-being.** Since yoga is beneficial to the mind, the body, and the spirit, you will begin to feel better in every way.

The Most Popular Types of Yoga

As explained earlier, there are many different types of yoga; and yoga isn't a religion. It is an approach to life. As such, it's very agile and flexible (no pun intended!) and carries well across cultural, country, and religious boundaries.

Thanks to its diversity, yoga has spread very swiftly throughout the western world over the last century; and it is now more and more popular among people of all ages - from children to elderly men and women - who want to improve their health and their life in general.

If you have experienced yoga in the past or seen it on television and felt it wasn't for you - or that you didn't like it at all, there is a good chance you weren't exposed to the right type of yoga.

Many think that if they've seen or experienced one type of yoga, they have seen it all. This is far from the truth.

People practice many different styles of yoga. Even though all types of yoga were developed from the same physical positions (poses), each type focuses on a particular situation.

Let's take a closer look at each type and its benefits to help you make a decision on which one is right for you.

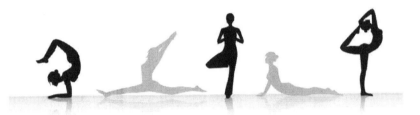

Hatha Yoga

Considered to be the most popular form of yoga in Western Society, Hatha yoga is practiced for both health and vitality, according to Graham Ledgerwood, teacher of yoga and mysticism for 30 years.

Ledgerwood states that Hatha Yoga is a "marvelous means of exercising, stretching, and freeing the body so it can be a healthy, long-lived, and vital instrument of the mind and soul."

The reason behind its popularity in Western Society, particularly in the United States, is that aside from being easy to learn, it is a good form of exercise and stress management.

It is recommended for beginners because the whole routine is slow-paced and provides a good foundation of basic yoga poses that preapre people for more complicated forms of yoga.

Hatha, a term derived from the Sanskrit term "Ha", is a form of yoga that is believed to be the foundation of all yoga styles.

It involves learning postures (Asanas), regulated breathing (Pranayama), meditation (Dharana & Dhyana) and Kundalini (Laya yoga) into a full system that is used by many individuals to obtain enlightenment and self-realization.

As with any other form of yoga, the easiest way to practice Hatha Yoga is to keep a clear mind and a relaxed body throughout your practice session. Take the time to meditate for a few minutes to achieve a peaceful state before you begin.

Once you are free of distractions, perform the poses with control and grace. You can go as long as you please but be sure that you don't overdo the asanas.

The main objectives of Hatha Yoga are:

1. **To meditate.** The art of learning to enter a meditative state is one of the most important aspects of yoga. In the beginning it is important to find a comfortable position that you can stay in for long periods of time to help you meditate. As you progress, you can add more variety in your meditative positions to allow yourself to go into even deeper concentration.

2. **To renew your body's energies and to reach optimum health.** After a long, tiring day, the objective of Hatha Yoga is to do stretches and various poses to help relax the body and to relieve it of stress

Ashtanga Yoga

Compared to Hatha, Ashtanga is a form of yoga that is more physically demanding. The name Ashtanga means "eight limbs" in Sanskrit and was derived from Sri K. Pattanhi Jois.

This form of yoga involves progressive and continuous asanas in the same order and moving from one position to another, which is referred to as 'flow' in yoga terminology.

As a result, the Ashtanga Yoga workout brings about intense internal heat as well as profuse, purifying sweat that help detoxify internal organs and muscles.

In order to successfully perform Ashtanga Yoga asanas, it is vital to master breathing techniques that will synchronize with the physical demands of the workout.

This form of yoga is not recommended for beginners; it is usually practiced by athletes and physically active individuals.

Some benefits of Ashtanga Yoga are:

- Better blood circulation
- Improved flexibility
- Improved stamina
- A lighter but stronger body
- A calm mind

Power Yoga

Basically a form of yoga with brawn, power yoga is believed to be the Americanized version of Ashtanga Yoga – only a little more complex and physical.

Power Yoga is a combination of stretching, strength training, and meditative breathing. Like an intense aerobic workout, many of the exercises performed resemble basic calisthenics such as push-ups, handstands, toe touches, and side bends.

The goal of Power Yoga is to work up a sweat and to build muscle which is why it's not a form of yoga recommended to first-timers or those who are recovering from an injury.

Ananda Yoga

Unlike the two previous forms of yoga, Ananda Yoga is not a physical workout. It focuses on gentle postures which are designed to move the energy from your body up to the brain in order to prepare your whole body for meditation.

Body alignment and controlled breathing are also practiced in Ananda Yoga. It teaches you how to harmonize the three most vital parts of your being – your mind, your body, and your spirit.

Beginners can try their hand at Ananda Yoga. Even though it does not require a physical workout, it does get more challenging as you gain more experience.

- Different aspects that Ananda Yoga focuses on:
- Learning safe and correct body alignment
- Maintaining a constant state of relaxation
- Adapting to poses that meet the needs of the practitioner

Anusara Yoga

Anusara is relatively a new form of yoga founded in 1997 by John Friend. The practice is based on the philosophy of "belief in the intrinsic goodness of all beings". That is why it is involves strict principles of alignment combined with a playful spirit.

The main focus of Anusara Yoga is to open your heart and connect with the Divine within you, as well as with the others around you.

Beginners and experienced practitioners alike can practice Anusara Yoga because it involves both light-hearted and challenging poses.

The poses are designed to be heart-oriented so you will have a deep feeling of connection inside, instead of trying to control your mind and body from the outside.

The art of Anusara Yoga is about co-participation with the Supreme and not trying to dominate, subjugate, or control nature. Its intention is to align with the Divine.

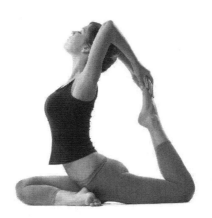

Bikram /Hot Yoga

Bikram Yoga was founded by 1963 Olympic weight lifting gold medalist Bikram Choudhury, hence the name. It is also referred to as hot yoga. The poses and exercises involved with this form of yoga are usually performed in a heated environment where the temperature can reach 95°-105° F.

Why 105 Degrees?

Based on Hatha Yoga poses and postures that help detoxify the body, Bikram is a form of yoga that also helps flush out waste products and toxins from your organs and glands.

At the same time it nourishes every cell of your body and offers a smooth, natural irrigation of your body through your circulatory system.

Bikram Yoga involves 26 poses which systematically work the whole body – each having a specific connection to different internal organs, blood vessels, ligaments, and muscles to achieve optimum health and maximum capacity.

By integrating heat into these poses, Bikram Yoga improves the process of detoxification. The heat also improves a practitioner's flexibility and helps to avoid injuries.

In addition, the comprehensive Bikram Yoga combines all elements and components of a good workout which includes the following

- Muscular strength
- Muscular endurance
- Cardiovascular flexibility
- Weight loss

Bikram is the only type of yoga that requires a specialized heated room for practice. It is not recommended for beginners; and, if you do practice Bikram, be sure you do so under the strict supervision of a certified Bikram Yoga instructor.

Integral Yoga

Integral Yoga is a simple form of yoga that aims for the practitioners to get in touch with their inner-selves, discover the strength that comes from the Divine, and to go on a journey to find themselves.

It is a meditative practice that focuses on synthesizing various branches and aspects of yoga.

It combines several yoga components such as

- Postures
- Breathing exercises
- Selfless service
- Meditation
- Chanting
- Prayer
- Self-inquiry

ISHTA Yoga

ISHTA, which stands for Integral Science of Hatha, Tantra, and Ayurveda, is a particular form of yoga developed by a South African teacher named Mani Finger. It was his son, Alan, that introduced the practice to the United States.

In Sanskrit, the name means "individual" and this is exactly the main focus of ISHTA yoga. The practice aims for its practitioners to accept and be comfortable with who they are and how they look.

ISHTA yoga involves various postures, visualizations, and meditation techniques that help the practitioners open their energy channels throughout their entire body.

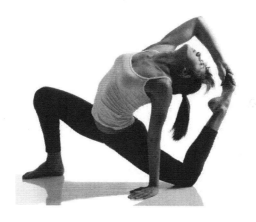

Iyengar Yoga

Iyengar yoga was initially developed in the 1950's by yoga master B.K.S. It remains to be one of the most popular types of yoga taught and practiced today.

What sets Iyengar Yoga apart from other forms is the requirement to use accessories and equipment such as mats, cushions, blankets, and straps during sessions.

These accessories help make the practice easier and more accessible to people, even those who are sick, old, disabled, or those who simply have a difficulty with flexibility.

Iyengar Yoga involves poses and postures that promote strength, flexibility, endurance, balance, and proper body alignment.

In this form of yoga, postures need to be held a little bit longer than in other types of yoga, and requires proper rest and breathingin between the postures..

All the poses, which come from the much broader style of yoga, Hatha Yoga (which is yoga's most basic form), are incorporated into Iyengar.

Iyengar Yoga is preferred by those who are recovering from an injury because of its slow pace and attention to detail.

Jivamukti Yoga

Jivamukti Yoga was developed in 1984 by Sharon Gannon and David Life, incorporating their study of Ashtanga Yoga and combining it with spiritual teachings while also putting special emphasis on how one can apply yogic philosophy to their daily life.

The name Jivamukti means "liberation while living" in Sanskrit and that is what you're in for once you try this form of yoga. Jivamukti can be aggressive and quite intense; perfect for those who are looking for a great workout.

Each class starts with a theme for the whole routine involving chanting, meditation, asana, pranayama, and music.

Hollywood stars like Gwyneth Paltrow, Russel Simmons and Sting are practitioners of Jivamukti yoga. so if you decide to attend a class, don't be surprised if you find yourself next to one of the big Hollywood stars!

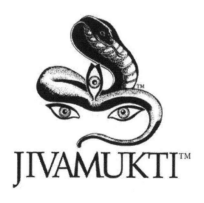

Kali Ray Triyoga

This particular form of yoga was developed by a great woman and yoga master, Kali Ray in 1980. The main aim of Kali Ray Triyoga is to take you on a real journey "into the flow," which is yoga terminology.

This can be done by incorporating a series of flowing, dance-like movements and postures, pranayama, and meditation.

In a single session of Kali Ray Triyoga, a practitioner will experience warm-up exercises leading to a workout, which isfollowed by meditation.

The meditation process involves deep relaxation by performing sustained asanas and flowing with the use of rhythmic breathing and a meditative mind.

The main aim of the Kali Ray Triyoga is to achieve strength and stillness for your inner self and for your true nature.

Kripalu Yoga

Kripalu Yoga is also known by the name of *Yoga of Consciousness.*

This is a gentle and introspective type of yoga which teaches the students to hold poses for longer periods of time so they can explore and release any emotional and spiritual blockages they might have.

Unlike other yoga styles, you don't have to achieve perfect alignment of your body nor do you have to be goal-oriented and strive to achieve a certain goal.

Kripalu Yoga consists of three phases or stages.

Stage One

This stage is about learning the various postures of Kripalu and exploring the practitioner's ability and limits in doing these postures.

Stage Two

Once you've learned the postures, you can move on to the second stage. In this stage you will learn to hold the postures for an extended period of time to increase concentration and inner awareness.

Stage Three

This stage takes some time to master as you learn to shift from one posture to another while in the meditative state. The movement from each position should arise unconsciously and spontaneously, letting you focus on things that are more important such as your breath, keeping your balance, and relaxation.

By practicing these type of postures everyday you will feel your blockages starting to dissolve, energy being released, and the healing process taking place on all levels. You will encounter and set free layers of stress, pain, and resistance that is lodged in your body without your even knowing it.

It will help you naturally accelerate the healing process and enable you to reach higher levels of emotional stability, you will be more clear mentally and will achieve a state of physical well-being.

Kripalu Yoga is aimed to work on your muscular-skeletal systems as well as your digestive, circulatory, respiratory, nervous, and immune systems.

Physical benefits of the Kripalu yoga are:

- Reduced anxiety
- Lower stress levels
- Lower blood pressure
- Increased relaxation
- Increased flexibility of your body
- Increased strength
- Higher endurance
- Increased levels of energy

In addition to the physical benefits, Kripalu Yoga sessions will have a pronounced effect on your mind and emotions as well.

Kripalu yoga is basically a tool for personal growth and empowerment

By practicing this type of yoga you will reach into your inner-knowing and learn how to become independent from external authorities. You will learn ways to be open to what others around you have to offer without losing your power to reason and to make your own decisions.

What is more important is that you will establish and create a strong, intimate, and nurturing relationship with your body.

In each session you transform your body into a temple in which you invite the presence of the Divine. This single intention can and will carry you to new depths in your practice and in life.

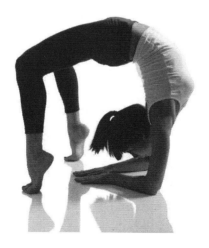

Kundalini Yoga

Known as the "yoga of awareness," Kundalini Yoga combines the three most important elements – physical, mental, and spiritual – which is why it is considered to be a special type of yoga.

Both the meditation and the kriyas in the practice of Kundalini are designed to raise complete body awareness and to prepare the body, nervous system, and mind to handle the energy of the Kundalini as it rises.

The main focus of Kundalini is to develop and improve your strength, awareness, consciousness, and your character. It also focuses on expanding sensory awareness and intuition with the purpose of raising personal consciousness and combining it with the infinite consciousness of God.

Most of the physical poses in Kundalini concentrate on navel and spine activity as well as selective pressurization of body points and meridians.

Through breathing exercises and the use of bhandas (three yogic locks) you are able to release, direct, and control how the Kundalini energy flows within your body – from the lower center, which is at the base of the spine, to the higher energetic center, which is in the head.

A special breathing technique that involves alternating the left and the right nostril is taught, along with the many meditations, kriyas, and practices of Kundalini Yoga. This is done in order to cleanse the nadis (subtle channels and pathways) to aid in awakening the Kundalini energy.

Restorative Yoga

This particular style of yoga focuses on using restful postures to completely relax your body. Do not confuse the term "rest" with sleep. Rest provides your body the chance to renew and heal itself from the inside.

Benefits of Restorative Yoga are that it can . . .

- Trigger the Parasympathetic Nervous System also known as the PNS. This is responsible for keeping your body in balance

- Lower heart rate

- Lower blood pressure

- Stimulate the immune system

- Keep the endocrine system functioning properly

To achieve deep relaxation of your body, Restorative Yoga makes use of different props and accessories. Using cushions or blocks makes it much easier for your body to get into certain postures and maintain that posture for longer periods of time. It is a way of surrendering.

Essential props include:

- Yoga block

- Yoga strap

- Blankets

- Yoga bolster

- Balls
- Chairs
- Wall
- Sandbags

You can practice Restorative Yoga any time of the day; but, one recommendation is that you start your day with yin poses and breathing exercises.

Also recommended is to practice restorative poses at the end of a long, busy day, before you go to sleep. This will help you sleep better and sustain higher levels of energy throughout the day.

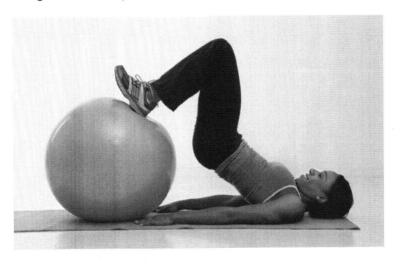

Moksha Yoga

Moksha Yoga is a relatively new form of yoga founded by yoga masters Ted Grant and Jessica Robertson in Toronto Canada in 2004.

Sometimes referred to as Moksha Hot Yoga, its popularity has increased quickly in the few years since its introduction.More and more studios have opened all over the world, including Canada, the United States, the Caribbean, and Switzerland.

The practice of Moksha Yoga is similar to Bikram because it involves the use of a hot room during a session. Like Bikram, it has several poses (about 40) which are designed to eliminate toxins from your body, to cleanse the body and mind, and to support life-long health.

Moksha Yoga is a combination of accessibility and challenge. Beginners can try their hands at this form of yoga if they can stand the heat.

Sivananda Yoga

Sivananda is similar to Hatha, only a more gentle version that focuses on the practitioner's overall health and wellness. Unlike aggressive and physically demanding forms of yoga such as Ashtanga and Vinyasa, Sivananda Yoga is the exact opposite. It only involves full yogic breathing and frequent relaxation.

The practice is not for athletes and physically active individuals but rather for those who want to de-stress.

Aside from relaxation, Sivananda Yoga sessions also work on the vitality of the body while decreasing the chances of certain diseases and illnesses.

The five core principles of Sivananda Yoga:

- Proper exercise: asanas
- Proper breathing: pranayama
- Proper Relaxation: sayasana
- Proper thinking and meditation
- Proper diet: vegetarian

A yogic, vegetarian diet is recommended throughout your sessions.

You are limited to sattvic food which includes:

- Water
- Cereal grains
- Mung beans
- Fruits
- Vegetables
- Nuts
- Un-pasteurized and un-homogenized milk
- Milk derivatives (mostly ghee, but also butter, cream, cheese, and yogurt)
- Raw honey

Svaroopa Yoga

Svaroopa is primarily recommended for beginners because its technique cannot be called an exercise, but rather an activity that focuses on deep, supported poses for spinal release.

The aim of Svaroopa Yoga is to keep the spine open while performing different techniques of precise alignment in poses that were selected very carefully.

These poses, combined with the right props placed meticulously in key points, will help you open up even the deepest tensions of the body. Sessions usually start with performing comfortable chair poses.

Svaroopa is an approachable style of yoga and is recommended for beginners. Svaroopa intermediate and advanced classes are available for different levels of ability and experience.

Viniyoga

The name Viniyoga is associated with numerous definitions. In Sanskrit, the name literally means "separation," "detachment," and "leaving." Other common meanings include "employment," "use." and "application."

Viniyoga is a therapeutic form of yoga, which is why it is recommended to people who have suffered an injury or who are recovering from surgery. It is also a good practice to help ease pain, as well as improve function in patients with chronic lower back pain.

Viniyoga is a very gentle form of yoga and is considered to be a healing practice tailored to each person's body type and needs

Vinyasa Yoga

Viniyasa yoga focuses on coordination of breath and movements.

This is a very physically active form of yoga; so, it is not recommended for individuals who suffer from any form of injury or who are not very active or mobile in their day to day life.

White Lotus Yoga

Developed by Ganga White, White Lotus is a modified version of Ashtanga Yoga. It is the combination of breathing techniques and meditation that aims to achieve inner peace and relaxation.

Yin Yoga

The sessions of Yin Yoga involve holding each pose for several minutes at a time because it aims to stretch the connective tissues around the joints.

The practice of Yin Yoga revolves around the belief that if you sit still and maintain a certain position for an extended period of time, you will gain therapeutic benefits for your connective tissues and not your muscles

Final Recommendations

The art and practice of yoga can be mastered over time. Keeping in mind what yoga is and isn't will take you a long way in the practice; and may eventually inspire you to help someone else.

Everyone and anyone can be a yoga teacher, with or without the presence of certification.

Regardless of the amount of knowledge you have, someone can still benefit from what you have learned through your personal experience.

One of the philosophies of yoga is, "Your teacher is within yourself."

All the teachings are universal, available for everybody. When faced with doubt, simply return to basics.

About the Author

Michelle Nicole is a thirty three year old free spirit who loves sleeping in on Sunday mornings or running barefoot on the beach. But above all, she is passionate about staying fit and healthy as well as helping others do the same.

She first began practicing yoga more than a decade ago. And is excited to share with others the knowledge she has gathered about yoga through her personal experience.

To find out more about Michelle Nicole and her other yoga books, visit her author's page on Amazon:

www.amazon.com/author/michellenicole